Also by Sheila Markstrom

BOLD STEPS DIET & FITNESS COMMITMENT JOURNAL

WORDS... Cause a Positive Ripple Effect

TRY AGAIN!

DON'T GIVE UP: The bold steps I took to lose 200 pounds for good.

Sheila Markstrom

TRY AGAIN! Don't give up: The bold steps I took to lose 200 pounds for good.

Copyright © 2016 by Sheila Markstrom

Library of Congress Control Number: 2015921092
Published by Markstrom Management, LLC, dba Bold Steps
Peoria, AZ

ISBN: 978-0-692-59855-9

Manufactured in the United States

To my family and friends, thank you for your heartfelt praise and support which was a significant contribution to reaching my weight loss goals.

To my brother, Scott, I am grateful for your suggestion and encouragement to share my weight loss journey inspiring and motivating others to pursue and achieve their goals.

With much appreciation and affection to Melissa, Barb, Scott, Linda, Margaret, Rhonda and Paige for providing excellent advice. I am grateful for your expertise, support and generosity.

Every accomplishment begins with a decision to try.

Edward T. Kelly

Table of Contents

The positive thinker sees the invisible, feels the intangible and achieves the impossible.

Anonymous

Introduction

How do those pounds keep coming back? They are like a boomerang, you work hard to shed them and without effort, they return.

Why do some of us struggle to lose weight? We start with good intentions but end in defeat. How do we change course... can we change course?

Yes, we can change course. We can choose to make permanent lifestyle changes. We can change our eating habits and we can change our level of fitness, but there are no short cuts. Learning to live a healthier life takes planning and dedication.

This is an account of how I finally succeeded in shedding 200 pounds after many years of losing the same battle again and again.

To begin let me provide a summary of my weight-centric history.

I have struggled with weight issues my whole life, well, except at birth. I came into the world just under 5 pounds and those first weeks are the only ones where I was underweight (and the only time I wore a size small!). What happened, how did I go so far off track?

When did my brain determine that I would "feel" better if I ate sweets? A brownie is not a substitute for a hug or a kind word, nor does it improve one's self-esteem.

I had several periods of weight loss achievement over the years but it never lasted more than a few months to a year before my emotions got in the way, derailing permanent success. You know the emotions: stress, sadness, loss, hurt, frustration, anger, depression, boredom, all the negative emotions. Of course I ate for positive reasons, too, celebrating achievements, activities and events.

Like many emotional eaters, carrot sticks and apples weren't what I reached for to squash the negative feelings. Stressed about work, I ate cookies. Nervous about a presentation, I ate candy. Anxiety over a deadline, I ate bagels. Concerned for a loved one, I ate chips. Hurt feelings, I ate ice cream. Depressed, I ate chocolate.

My reactions to the emotional triggers were on autopilot, they never changed. Why did I always reach for and devour candy, ice cream or cookies? The sugar demons were always in motion and my willpower was MIA.

When you are wallowing in negative emotions do you sometimes wonder how that empty bag of peanut M&M's got in your hands, realizing you've consumed a bag, only after every piece is gone? I've done that on more than one occasion. At those times it was as if my subconscious was a separate entity with no empathy. With my realization came the guilt, the shame and the negative self-talk, "What's wrong with me?", "I am fat and getting fatter!", "I hate the way I look, why can't I fix this?"... "I am unlovable."

Would I ever be able to make a permanent change after years, decades, of emotional binge eating?

As odd as this sounds, yet, it may make sense to some - I hid behind the weight. It was my reason, my excuse or what I blamed to avoid facing problems, challenges, and reality. A bit crazy, I know. I desperately wanted to lose the weight and end the downward spiral but I sabotaged myself at every turn.

The conflict in my brain raged on. I knew what to do. I wanted to do it. Why did my subconscious undermine my efforts and how would I break through?

In moments of clarity I would get on track but only with short-lived success. Losing weight was a never-ending battle of unsustainable effort followed by regretful and depressing binge eating which was, of course, followed by the inevitable weight-gain.

During my early to late 20's my weight fluctuated by 10-25 pounds above average. Then from my late 20's to late-30's I grappled with self-doubt issues and depression, a turbulent period, resulting in my weight jumping from 150 pounds to over 300 pounds.

300 pounds became the new normal.

This new normal led to the weight-gain – weight-loss – weight-gain cycle playing over and over, again.

A historical look (with total vulnerability) at my major weight loss attempts:

- **Age: 42 / Weight: 307**

    I lost 129 pounds in 15 months and was 28 pounds from my goal. Then I hit a difficult period that challenged my self-esteem, again. I completely misjudged a personal relationship which affected my confidence and hit me financially.

    Overwhelmed, I reverted back to my old ways. No matter how many pints of ice cream I stacked around me, I couldn't consume enough to build a level of euphoria, to camouflage the self-doubt and disillusionment.

    My weight loss method had been misguided and unsustainable. My calorie intake was well below acceptable numbers and the exhausting hours of daily exercise I fit in around a 60 hour work week was impossible to maintain. I gained the 129 pounds plus 33 more in half the time it took to lose it. I weighed 340 pounds.

    There were a few minor attempts in the following years, then...

- Age: 51 / Weight: 340

I lost 125 pounds in 15 months but this time I was 65 pounds from my goal when I took on new work responsibilities increasing my schedule to 70+ hours per week and doubling my business travel frequency.

My career had always been a significant part of who I am, it provided the opportunity to prove my capabilities, my value and to be accepted. Place that against my self-esteem issues, and my emotional eating addiction, and it's easy to see the correlation to constant weight battles.

My weight loss methods had been the same as before – unsustainable. I was consuming just 500-1,000 total calories per day and exercising up to 3 hours every day. I regained the 125 pounds in record time.

The pattern of minor weight loss success, followed by regaining the weight continued, until...

At my largest I weighed a shocking and depressing 372 pounds.

Revelation: in my third attempt to lose over 100 pounds (in reality, now over 200 pounds) and to have enduring success I had to approach this overwhelming goal in a permanent life changing way. I needed to take bold steps, not crazy steps but smart, bold steps.

No more drastic measures that don't work for the long term, no more unhealthy 500 calorie days. No more 3 hour daily exercise routines that I couldn't maintain.

While surgery, fad diets and shakes are a choice for some, they weren't for me. My history had proven that there was no easy and fast way to lose this much weight and keep it off for good. It may seem like I gained 200 pounds overnight but in reality it took time to put all the weight on and it would take time to take it all off.

I had lived a lifetime of eating to soothe my negative emotions. I needed to accomplish my weight loss goal in a way that would mean:

- A change to how I dealt with those emotions
- A change to how I viewed my self-image and worth
- A change to how I approached my relationship with food
- A change in my lax commitment to regular exercise

What made the difference for me this time and how would I achieve lasting success? I thought about the "why" I ate and the "what" I ate and the "when" I ate. And, I thought about what needed to change in my head to get to a new healthy reality.

From this starting point I executed a plan incorporating the following essential elements:

Forgiveness

Attitude

Commitment

Strategy

Motivation

Fortitude

Celebration

Gratitude

This challenge was by far the most difficult and frustrating challenge of my life. This journey wasn't easy and I had a few missteps along the way, but I was determined to take bold steps and **try again**.

Listen, I am not a medical professional and I would encourage you to see one as I did during my weight loss journey. This is a personal account of my struggles, strategy and ultimate success at achieving weight and fitness improvement goals. I hope that my story will inspire and motivate you to reach your goals.

Who you are tomorrow begins with what you do today.

Tim Fargo

Chapter 1

Why Now?

You know the saying: "Live your best life" - I wanted to do just that. It was time to push past the emotional roadblocks and to discard the shield of fat I hid behind. It was time to move forward. Only I could change my future.

Again, why now?

No Energy

- I was tired
- I was lethargic
- I quit participating in activities I used to enjoy
- I was existing but not truly living

Embarrassment

It happened on a business trip. The first thing one does when we settle into an airplane seat is fasten the seat belt. But this time no matter how hard I tried, no matter how hard I squeezed in my gut I couldn't get the seatbelt to close. I had to ask a flight attendant for a seat belt extension; she wasn't discreet in giving me one and everyone nearby noticed. Total humiliation.

This is just one of the many embarrassing moments I had with my huge size, there were so many more:

- Walking into a room, an office, a restaurant, a theater and worrying about being able to fit into a chair
- Knowing I was the fattest person in a room full of people... nowhere to hide
- Seeing friends and business associates that hadn't seen me since gaining (or regaining) a huge amount of weight
- As a frequent business traveler – the dreaded small plane seats (would the next flight be the one that someone complained about me sitting next to them?)
- Clothes shopping – no matter how much I spent on good quality clothing I couldn't hide my rolls of fat
- Grocery shopping – I shopped at 6 am on the weekend to avoid shoppers peering into my basket and thinking "why is that fat women buying ice cream"
- Participating in sports – bending, squatting, jumping, running had all become impossible to do
- Climbing stairs – barely making it to the top and then being out of breathe for several minutes and unable to hold a conversation
- Retrieving something I dropped on the floor – hoping no one was watching as I struggled to bend over and pick it up
- Thigh friction – the noise made when pant legs rub together
- Turning down invitations worrying that I wouldn't "fit" in – never explaining the real reason for the decline which unintentionally hurt friend's feelings
- Dating – closing myself off, I was too fat, I wasn't going to set myself up for the inevitable rejection
- Business presentations with all eyes on me

- Refusing to let anyone take my picture – did I really think someone wouldn't remember how fat I was if they didn't have a photo?
- Doctor appointments, and worse, the dreaded scale!
- The list is endless

Depression

- The insurmountable goal of losing 200 pounds
- Ashamed that I hadn't succeeded in the past
- Always feeling self-conscious by how I looked
- Hiding from my life

My Health

I was told that if I didn't lose weight immediately a diabetic diagnosis was inevitable. For me, this was a serious scare that could further damage my eye sight. I had been diagnosed with severe Glaucoma two years earlier, a result of chronic Uveitis (inflammation). Glaucoma can be a complication of diabetes and it is a leading cause of blindness.

My biological mother had died of complications from diabetes at age 72. She had also lost her eye sight. Was this my future? It was hard to believe that the only thing I might inherit from the woman I'd seen once since I was five years old would be diabetes and blindness. As if dealing with a lifetime of self-doubt wasn't enough. I was scared but this, too, was another life challenge to conquer.

It was a major wake-up call! No more games, no more guilt, no more self-criticism. I needed to make significant and permanent changes to my diet and fitness level immediately.

That is an easy statement to make but to create a plan, put it into action and to follow-through would take:

- Forgiving myself for past defeats
- Figuring out how to deal with negative emotions without turning to food
- Moving forward with a positive and accepting spirit
- Determining my specific weight loss goal
- Developing a healthy food and fitness strategy to reach my goal
- Determination, hard work and perseverance for the length of time it would take to achieve my goal
- A circle of family and friends that believed in me
- Rewarding achievements
- Courage

You have probably heard or read ads that state:

"You can eat whatever you want and still lose weight"...
"Lose weight fast/the pounds will melt right off"...
"Losing weight is easier than you think"... or "Lose weight without changing your lifestyle."

We know the reality, losing weight is not easy. If it were, none of us would be overweight. Without making lifestyle changes any weight loss achieved cannot be sustained permanently.

What does being "physically fit" mean to me? I wasn't born to be a 5'8", 125 pound, size 6 woman. And I am okay with that. As important as being physically fit is, what goes on in my brain and heart is essential. I want to be physically fit so that I can enjoy every aspect of my life for as long as is meant to be.

While I determined an approximate weight as my goal I knew that it would be the combination of feeling healthy, getting good numbers from the Doctor (blood pressure, cholesterol, etc.) and being able to actively participate in and enjoy life that would result in my ultimate success.

This is where my challenge began, starting with forgiveness.

Every moment in life, including
this one, is a fresh start.

R.J. Marshal

Chapter 2

Forgiveness

Forgiveness takes kindness, empathy and love. Why is it so difficult to forgive ourselves for things we wouldn't hesitate to forgive and provide comfort for with others? We can be incredibly hard on ourselves resulting in a variety of negative responses and actions.

To begin this journey, self-forgiveness was paramount to taking the first step, keeping on track, and achieving success. I needed to forgive myself for my past failed weight-loss attempts. I needed to forgive myself for all of the self-criticism and self-doubt, and most important, I needed to forgive and accept me inside and out.

This effort was all about the "stuff" buried deep and tied to my self-esteem. When would I decide I was good enough, that I deserved better for myself, and that I was worthy? It was time to untether the weight of all my emotional baggage.

While a couple of rounds of therapy over the years had moved me in the right direction, I hadn't taken the final steps. That would take self-reflection, self-compassion and self-acceptance.

I was ready.

To make clear and give impact to my self-forgiveness I decided to write my words down and create a *Forgiveness Impact Statement*. I wanted to force the pain out onto paper and honor myself with the forgiveness I deserved, to move past the self-criticism and the wall of fat.

My Forgiveness Impact Statement:

I forgive my past unsuccessful weight-loss attempts.
I forgive my past inability to sustain a long-term
commitment to exercise.
I forgive my constant self-criticism and self-doubt.
I forgive the past life challenges that have stopped
me from loving myself.
I am a good soul worthy of love.

This was a huge step. Insert big self-hug here with a smile. I was ready to begin my weight loss journey.

Attitude is a little thing that makes a big difference.

Winston Churchill

Chapter 3

Attitude

Funny thing about "attitude", we each have the power to change our negative attitude at any time and once we change our attitude, good things happen. Karma.

When we think positive, speak positive and do positive, we get more positive! It all starts with the brain and my brain needed an attitude adjustment in order to move past the emotional eating. I needed to eliminate my negative thoughts, "I'm fat", "I'll never lose the weight", and "I can't do it".

To move from a negative attitude about my self-image to a positive state of mind I first needed to forgive myself, as expressed in the previous chapter, and then accept myself. I continue to work on this daily and I am making progress.

To aid my change in attitude about my weight (and life in general) I decided to use mantras and affirmations to begin every day. I have several that I rotate and use. These mantras are typed and taped to my bathroom mirror. While looking in the mirror each morning I state one or more of the mantras out loud, sometimes all of them.

During the course of the day I will repeat one or more of the mantras for reinforcement.

My mantras:

- **Attitude is Everything – Pick a Good One!**
  Dr. Wayne Dyer

- *SMILE* ☺ (yes, there is a smiley face)

- **Be Joyful**

- **Change my mind. Change my body.**
  Ann Kearney-Cooke, Ph.D.

- *Today is a Good Day for a Good Day!*
  Heather Delany Reese

- *Focus on the solution, not the problem.*
  Walter Anderson

- *Eat Less + Move More = Weight Loss*

- *I like what I see!* ☺

- *Make Peace with Myself*

The hardest mantra for me to say and by far the most meaningful one is the last mantra above. Without internal peace I knew I couldn't permanently lose the weight. Internal peace was at the core of my weight "issues", my head and body connection.

Many of us have life experiences in childhood that formed specific responses to negative feelings/emotions that as adults still play over and over in our head. While I have no memories of my birth mother I have lived with the feeling of rejection, abandonment and being unlovable since she

28

walked out on us when I was five. Picture a five-year old little girl thinking "there must be something wrong with me if my mommy doesn't want me."

Compounding the feeling of not being wanted was my birth mother taking my 7-year old sister with her. In my 5-year old mind, "I must really be bad/unlovable if my mommy wants my sister but she doesn't want me." Years later when I was eighteen, while in conversation with a paternal aunt, I stated I never understood why my birth mother wanted my sister but not me. Shocker, I learned that this sister was not my Dad's daughter. Long before this revelation the damage had been done. Even though I was loved by my kind, caring and honorable Dad, my paternal Grandmother and Step-Mom, the feeling of worthlessness had always been too deep to shed.

I lived my life internally believing I was "not good enough".

The negative emotions derived from our past experiences can manifest in a variety of ways. In my case that has always meant unhealthy eating. At every turn food was my comfort. Knowing and understanding the reason I soothed emotional pain with food was key to my well-being. Breaking the emotional eating habit and altering my behavioral response to negative emotions had been my toughest challenge but it was time to change that. Starting with an optimistic attitude.

Accomplishing the essential element of changing my attitude would be the only way I could achieve lasting success.

Taking the last mantra above one step further I made a revision:

Forgive and Make Peace with Myself

Let me repeat... *Forgive and Make Peace with Myself*

Was it easy to repeat these mantras, from the start? No.

Did I initially state them every day? No, it was an adjustment.

In the beginning did I believe in the words for me? No, but I kept at it.

The more uncomfortable I felt the more I knew how important these mantras were to my mission. I knew if I continued with them the words would become real and meaningful. The mantras would help me achieve the positive attitude I needed to be successful in losing weight and, with time, the words did just that.

It is amazing how powerful this daily ritual has become.

How will you change your attitude to help work on your self-improvement efforts? If you decide to include your own mantras there are many websites online with inspirational quotes such as: quotes-inspirational.com, brainyquotes.com, and inspirationalquotes4u.com. Modify them or create your own. This action will move you in the right direction.

In addition, the adage, "Laughter is the best medicine" is true. *Lighten-up to lighten up.* (Another great mantra!)

While making these lifestyle changes was serious for me, I knew I needed to keep my sense of humor and let it loose more frequently. Laughter was a huge antidote to building my positive attitude.

Life is more fun, more enjoyable and more rewarding when we laugh.

Balance. In combination with reinforcing a positive attitude and letting in more laughter I needed to improve my life balance, the balance between work and personnel life.

My work life had always been the priority and my personal life suffered for it. When one is constantly at internal battle to work the hardest, do the most, be the best, be the first in and last to leave, trying to eliminate any potential for criticism or failure, there is no time, no energy, and no interest in exercise. Of course, for me, the added stress meant more out of control eating.

To be a success with my diet & fitness goals I needed to prioritize a healthy balance between work and my personal life. A balance I work at every day.

I have also worked on changing my "**shoulds**" to "**wants**" improving the odds of a positive outcome:

- "I should make healthier food choices" is now: "I want to make healthier food choices"
- "I should exercise" is now: "I want to exercise"
- "I should be more positive" is now: "I want to be / I am more positive"

Have you ever noticed that "shoulds" come with a frown while "wants" come with a smile? This simple word change has had a significant impact.

Great attitude.   More laughter.   Better life balance.

The discipline of writing something down is the first step toward making it happen.

Lee Iacoca

Chapter 4

Commitment

Knowing what I needed to do to lose weight wasn't the concern... we all know what we need to do:

- Eat Less   Consuming fewer calories each day will result in weight loss
- Eat Healthy   Eat lean protein and lots of veggies and fruit fueling my body with the healthiest calories
- Move More   Doing more cardio and eating fewer calories will result in weight loss
- Build Muscle   Lifting weights builds muscle – muscle burns more calories faster
- Hydrate   Water is a key ingredient for healthier living – drink up!
- Sleep   Get the 7-8 hours of sleep my body needs to be rejuvenated and refreshed every day
- Reduce Stress   Attitude adjustment and positive mantras will reduce stress and create a healthier environment
- Live Positive   My #1 factor for weight loss and exercise motivation

These actions are common sense but how do we get from knowing what to do to actually doing it?

Commitment.

We make a commitment.

I needed to have a clear and specific goal to commit to the herculean effort of losing 200 pounds. To commit to that goal I needed to write it down and make it real. I created a *Commitment Goal Statement.*

My objective was to write a goal statement that was realistic and achievable with hard work and dedication. A goal statement I could refer to, live by, and measure. Measurement would be crucial to maintaining my commitment throughout the journey and ultimately to reaching my goal.

My Commitment Goal Statement

With a positive attitude, a solid strategy for achieving diet & exercise improvement, and with unwavering perseverance - I will lose 200 pounds in three years. I will chart and monitor my actions to keep me on track to reaching my weight loss goal. Through this effort I will transition to living a healthy lifestyle.

How I determined the components of my goal statement:

- I would need to maintain a positive attitude to get started and to stay on course
- I needed to develop a diet and exercise strategy that would be key to achieving long-term success
- I would go through a variety of roadblocks as I worked to reach my goal. It would take determination and resolve to keep on track – perseverance

- I would need to allow a realistic period of time to achieve success. Ultimately I wanted to lose 222 pounds but I was told by my physicians' assistant that the last 20-30 pounds would be very difficult to lose as the weight would primarily be the lose skin that I couldn't get rid of without surgery. Yuck! ...but I am trying!

Take to heart from my experience, the younger you are when you get your excess weight off and, if you include strength training in the process, the less likely chance that your skin won't contract. Alas, some drooping skin is far better than rolls of fat!

- I needed to chart and monitor my diet and exercise activity throughout this journey so that I could analyze any changes needed to achieve success

With my goal statement done I typed it up and signed it to strengthen my commitment. Then I printed several copies to keep in various places: taped to the refrigerator, taped to the bathroom mirror, in the nightstand, in my purse, in my briefcase and pinned to my office wallboard. I wanted to keep the goal in sight. I also stated my goal out loud repeatedly (like the mantras) for added emphasis and to help transition to my new healthy mindset.

I created a second goal statement shown in Chapter 11 – *Healthy Lifestyle Achieved.* Reaching my goal of losing 200 pounds was part one of two parts. In part two, I wanted to commit to maintaining my weight loss and improved fitness long-term.

Have you set a goal for yourself? To make it a reality create your own *Commitment Goal Statement* determining the elements needed to achieve success. Write it down and sign it, this is your starting point and your foundation.

Today is your day. To start fresh. To eat right.
To train hard. To live healthy. To be proud.

Bonnie Pfiester

Chapter 5

Strategy

For me it would require a balanced and multi-faceted strategy to achieve weight loss success. A strategy that would transform my poor eating and exercise habits into health-conscious living.

Plain and simple... I needed to burn more calories than I consumed every day. To get more detailed though, the components of my strategy are outlined on the following pages which include:

Step 1	Forgiveness & Peace
Step 2	Make Healthy Food Choices
Step 3	Incorporate Daily Exercise
Step 4	Practice Positive Self-Talk
Step 5	Educate & Equip
Step 6	Manage Social Events
Step 7	Emotional Trigger Solutions
Step 8	Support
Step 9	Accountability

What components will you put together to form the strategy to achieve your goal?

EAT LESS + MOVE MORE = WEIGHT LOSS

Note: A reminder – I am not a medical professional. Please consult with your Doctor, as I did, before embarking on your diet and exercise plan.

Strategy - Step 1

Forgive & Make Peace

No more obsessing about the past.

Yes, I had yo-yo dieted for years losing one battle after another. Yes, I had lost 125 and 129 pounds on previous attempts only to gain it all back and then some, getting fatter with each decade.

That is history and history serves as knowledge. That knowledge was the basis for making improvements to my previously unsuccessful weight loss attempts.

Forgive

As stated in chapter 2, forgiveness would be paramount if I was to achieve weight loss success. I forgave myself for failing at previous attempts and I applauded myself for trying. I forgave my negativity and self-deprecation.

Without forgiveness I would constantly look back and worry that I would end with the same past result, defeat. A defeatist attitude is not the best way to build momentum.

With forgiveness I could look back and determine what changes and enhancements I needed to make that would result in long-term success. With forgiveness I could move forward with positive energy and confidence. Smart!

Make Peace

An attitude adjustment, stating mantras plus adding meditation and deep breathing exercises, would all support my ability to achieve internal peace.

Making peace would improve my self-esteem, close the door on history and encourage my goal attainment. With a calm positive spirit – all good things are possible.

Forgive and make peace with myself, an easy concept in theory but far from easy to achieve after decades of self-abuse. With commitment and daily effort I have made significant strides toward this objective.

Work on forgiving yourself for past mistakes and setbacks. Without forgiveness your target is unattainable.

EAT LESS + MOVE MORE = WEIGHT LOSS

Strategy - Step 2

Make Healthy Food Choices

What I know for sure is that reducing my caloric intake below 1,000 calories per day is not sustainable for the long-term and it's not healthy.

What I quickly learned as I began my weight loss challenge this time was that I was losing weight faster eating more calories than I did when I was starving myself. I just needed to eat the right calories! What was right for me was eating a healthy 1,200-1,500 calories per day, in agreement with my doctor.

To take a bold step down the right path to weight loss and healthy eating I made a list of tips that I followed and added to as I continued on my journey. I needed to take control of the hold certain foods had on my psyche by adhering closely to this list.

These tips were significant lifestyle changes that I knew would make a huge impact:

Diet Tips

#1   Drink more water – at least 7-8 glasses per day; ice cold water that may help burn calories

#2   Eat breakfast every day – and include a lean protein; hard-boiled eggs are my quick and easy go-to breakfast. Stay away from cereal and juice that have a lot of sugar.

#3   Eat 3 meals a day – making all calories count toward good health – no more empty calories

#4   Don't skip meals – it will only backfire

#5   Don't get on the scale every day – weigh once a week on the same day and at the same time. To keep positive I wanted to reduce the frequency of getting on the scale where I would see no loss; or worse a pound or two gain. It isn't easy to hold out but it is worth it for both body and mind. Once I reached my goal I knew it would be important to weigh myself more frequently to maintain my achievement.

#6   Eat slower – enjoy the food and feel the fullness before eating too much

#7   Be mindful of what I eat – are these calories healthy? Focus on the food I can eat not the food I shouldn't eat. Make the calories count!

#8   Before eating – ask myself if I am hungry or am I feeling strong emotions?

#9   Eat more fruit: blueberries, raspberries, strawberries, blackberries, apples, cherries, peaches, pears, nectarines, melons, grapes, bananas, grapefruit, oranges, pineapple, apricots, etc. (not fruit juice)

#10 Keep my fruit bowl full and on the kitchen counter for easy access and as a visual reminder of healthy snacks

#11 Eat more veggies: asparagus, broccoli, beets, squash, peppers, tomatoes, cauliflower, peas, onions, scallions, mushrooms, yams, green beans, etc. And greens: arugula, lettuce, spinach, romaine, cabbage, endive, radicchio, etc.

#12 Eat water-rich foods which will help me feel fuller while eating fewer calories: watermelon, cantaloupe, strawberries, grapefruit, tomatoes, lettuce, spinach, cucumbers, zucchini, peppers, cabbage, broccoli

#13 Eat lean protein – poultry, fish, lean cuts of meat, eggs, beans (red kidney, cannellini, black, pinto, great northern, navy), lentils, cheese, yogurt etc.

#14 Eat more raw/natural nuts and seeds: almonds, walnuts, macadamia nuts, pecans, pistachios, pumpkin seeds, sunflower seeds

#15 Eat more salmon (wild not farm-raised) – once a week or more

#16 Get enough fiber – eat whole grains like oats, couscous, brown rice, quinoa, barley, etc.

#17 Drastically reduce sugar consumption and don't use artificial substitutes

#18 Cut-out white bread, white rice and pasta (eat whole-grain equivalents)

#19 Eat fresh – no processed or refined packaged foods

#20 Don't keep sweets, ice cream or chips in the house (eliminate temptation)

#21 Use spices and herbs to flavor foods: cinnamon, vanilla, nutmeg, cardamom, turmeric, cayenne, garlic, pepper, ginger, cumin, onion, oregano, rosemary, basil, tarragon, thyme, seasoning blends, etc. Additional flavorings include vinegars (balsamic, apple cider, wine), fresh lemon, lime and orange juice, broth, low sodium soy sauce, worcestershire sauce, hot sauce, etc.

#22 Salsa is a great condiment for more than tortilla chips & tacos. It's fantastic on veggies, a bun-less veggie burger, a chicken breast, a baked potato, no-fat cottage cheese and more.

#23 Eat good fats in moderation – nuts, peanut butter, cheese, yogurt, avocados, etc.

#24 No fried foods – cook healthy: grill, broil, roast, steam, poach and stir-fry

#25 Use smaller dinner plates (or a salad plate) to shrink portions – visually a full plate while consuming fewer calories in total. Use a salad fork rather than a dinner fork to slow down so that I feel the fullness before eating more than I need.

#26 Control portions – an overflowing 1 cup measure is more than one cup! Same for a tablespoon! Don't eat from the package (bag/box); don't serve family style – plate food.

#27 Eat dairy products (Greek yogurt, no fat cottage cheese and milk/almond milk) in moderation but pay attention to the sugar content

#28 No junk food - have healthy snacks ready in individual servings: fruit, veggies, nuts, seeds, light cheese

#29 Track daily food intake: calories, fat, protein – use an online tool, an app or create a tracking chart (see example that follows *Tips*).

#30 When counting calories, add an extra 100 calories to the day's total for better accuracy against using my estimates

#31 Chew sugarless gum to avoid reaching for sweets

#32 Take a multi-vitamin daily (thankfully adult gummies were created!)

#33 Read food labels at the grocery store. Do not buy foods with high levels of sugar, fat or carbs. No trans fats, food coloring, artificial sweeteners, high-fructose syrup and other forms of sugar

#34 No soda (regular or diet), no juice, no sports drinks; cold ice water is my go-to beverage

#35 Limit alcohol to 1 glass of red wine 2-3 times a week

#36 Since I don't drink coffee or tea (never acquired a taste for either) I do allow myself a cup of hot cocoa on cold winter mornings

#37 Dark chocolate in moderation

#38 Use olive oil, canola oil, sesame oil, coconut oil (or similar) for cooking – no vegetable oil

#39 Stay away from cream-based entrees

#40 Don't eat meals sitting in front of the T.V. and turn the phone down or off

#41 Don't eat within 2.5-3 hours of bedtime or set a specific time each night that I stop eating

#42 Don't buy food in bulk – minimize temptation

#43 Out of reach, out of mind – stash food out of sight

#44 Plan ahead to eliminate last minute unhealthy meal choices

#45 Plan ahead for grocery shopping (build a list) and don't go shopping on an empty stomach

#46 Hit my local Farmers Market(s) for in-season fruits & veggies and specialty items

#47 Bring my lunch to work; don't eat lunch at my desk

#48 Limit cheat days – the potential for overindulgence is too great

#49 Don't eat the calories I just burned at the gym

#50 Be aware of people that may try to sabotage my efforts, nicely ask them to respect my decisions and goals; better yet, hang with like-minded, health & fitness conscious friends

#51 When I have friends or family over for a meal – send them home with any leftover dessert

#52 If eating dessert at a friend's home or a restaurant either politely decline the dessert or limit myself to just 2-3 bites

#53 Watch fewer cooking shows; restrain from reading magazines with lots of food photos – again, eliminate temptation

#54 Stop rewarding my behaviors, emotions, and wins/achievements with food

#55 Be patient, change takes time. Don't give up!

Tracking Calories

To keep disciplined and to achieve success I tracked all of my daily calories which included many healthy foods that I ate consistently:

Breakfast: hard-boiled eggs, omelet with veggies, oatmeal with fruit, English muffin with peanut butter, Greek yogurt & fruit

Lunch: tuna with chopped tomatoes, cucumbers and pickles (or with relish and no-fat cottage cheese), turkey slices with Swiss cheese and pickle on rye crisp, veggie burger (no bun) with a scoop of no-fat cottage cheese and salsa, Greek yogurt or non-fat cottage cheese and fresh fruit and/or nuts, a green salad with oil and balsamic vinegar or no dressing

Dinner: chicken or turkey & veggies, chicken & salad, chicken & beans with chopped tomatoes and salsa, fish & veggies, veggie burger (no bun) with a scoop of no-fat cottage cheese and salsa, shell fish & veggie kabobs, salad with oil and balsamic vinegar, or just veggies

Snacks: mixed berries, chopped apples with cinnamon, oranges, pineapple, melon and other fruits, frozen fruit bars (no added sugar), almonds, dried fruit, Greek yogurt with fruit, veggie sticks w/salsa, hardboiled eggs, no fat cottage cheese, grape tomatoes, smoothies, dark chocolate, low sugar trail mix or fruit & nut bars (no high sugar energy bars)

The following example of a food count chart tracks calories, fat and protein grams on a daily basis each month. I liked the process of filling-in the chart every day which reinforced my daily objectives with the diet.

There are many templates to use online and many apps to choose from or you can create your own chart, as I did.

EAT LESS + MOVE MORE = WEIGHT LOSS

Example of a Food Log

DAILY FOOD COUNT LOG   Month: October

C = Calories   F = Fat grams   P = Protein grams

Day	Breakfast C	F	P	Snack C	F	P	Lunch C	F	P	Snack C	F	P	Dinner C	F	P	Snack C	F	P	TOTALS C	F	P
1	120	8	12	160	14	6	260	1	38	115	1	1	450	15	36	210	6	8	1321	45	101
2	120	8	12	90	5	10	225	5	15	260	0	0	270	2	26	210	6	8	1175	25	71
3	120	8	12	160	14	6	310	1	33	210	0	0	303	2	33	170	5	8	1273	22	92
4	260	4	8	160	14	6	250	1	38	150	5	8	303	2	33	70	0	0	1193	26	93
5	120	8	12	160	14	6	205	5	15	70	0	0	510	8	28	240	4	0	1305	39	61
6	120	8	12	90	5	10	260	1	38	200	0	0	450	15	36	140	0	0	1260	28	96
7	120	8	12	120	0	0	225	5	15	120	0	0	356	2	42	170	5	8	1111	20	77
8	120	8	12	160	14	6	280	21	5	105	1	1	325	1	32	210	6	8	1200	51	64
9	260	4	8	120	0	0	260	1	38	140	0	0	450	15	18	140	0	0	1370	19	64
10	120	8	12	90	5	10	225	5	15	120	0	0	310	1	33	210	6	8	1075	24	78
11	120	8	12	160	14	6	260	1	38	150	5	7	325	1	32	170	5	8	1185	34	103
12	120	8	12	160	14	6	310	1	33	190	0	0	323	2	31				1103	24	82
13	120	8	12	160	14	6	225	5	15	70	0	0	705	6	31	310	6	2	1590	39	66
14	120	8	12	160	14	6	260	1	38	200	0	0	290	2	26	150	5	7	1180	29	89
15	210	13	22	70	0	0	280	21	5	120	0	0	450	15	36	180	0	2	1310	49	65
16	260	4	8	90	5	10	260	1	38	120	0	0	325	1	32	150	5	7	1205	15	95
17	120	8	12	160	14	6	225	5	15	210	0	0	323	2	33	210	6	8	1248	35	74
18	120	8	12	160	14	6	260	1	38	120	0	0	323	2	33	170	5	8	1153	30	97
19	210	13	22	70	0	0	225	5	15	120	0	0	320	4	21	200	0	1	1145	22	59
20	120	8	12	90	5	10	310	1	33	60	0	0	480	36	9	150	5	7	1210	54	71
21	120	8	12	90	5	10	280	21	5	60	0	0	303	2	33	250	6	10	1103	36	70
22	120	8	12	160	14	6	260	1	38	140	0	0	310	1	33	170	5	8	1160	28	97
23	210	13	22	160	14	6	225	5	15	115	1	0	306	2	42	210	6	8	1226	41	93
24	210	13	22	160	14	6	260	1	38	60	0	0	430	15	18	140	0	0	1260	42	84
25	260	4	8	120	8	6	260	1	38	200	0	0	290	2	28				1130	52	80
26	120	8	12	90	5	10	225	5	15	170	5	8	606	4	52	170	5	8	1381	32	105
27	120	8	12	260	4	8	280	21	5	115	1	0	325	1	32	210	6	8	1310	41	65
28	120	8	12	120	0	0	260	1	38	120	0	0	450	15	36	170	5	8	1240	29	94
29	120	8	12	160	14	6	225	5	15	120	0	0	310	1	33	150	5	7	1085	33	73
30	120	8	12	120	0	0	310	1	33	160	14	6	688	4	44				1398	27	95
31	120	8	12	90	5	10	260	1	38	120	0	0	303	2	33	210	6	8	1103	21	101

Average Per Day   Calories: 1226   Fat: 32.7   Protein: 82.4

51

Incorporate Daily Exercise

The greatest impact from my weight loss effort would be permanent change to my diet lifestyle. To enhance the results of this change I needed to (and wanted to) incorporate regular exercise.

Throughout my adult life I have always felt good when I exercised. Unfortunately I didn't maintain a consistent routine. Exercise commitment is an integral component of living a healthy life. I knew the benefits derived from a regular routine:

- Increased energy
- Reduced stress
- More confidence
- Reduced depression
- Better sleep
- Better focus and improved memory
- Keeps cognitive abilities sharp
- Reduced potential for illness
- Reduced inflammation
- More flexibility and balance
- Sense of accomplishment
- Satisfaction
- The happy – euphoric feeling

When my negative emotions were in full swing, when the unhealthy eating increased, my motivation to exercise shut down. When my motivation died the double whammy ensued:

Eat More + Move Less = <u>Weight Gain</u>!

A regular exercise routine as part of my weight loss strategy was imperative for success. I would make exercise part of my healthy permanent lifestyle change by incorporating a variety of physical activities that would enhance my overall fitness capability and reduce the potential for burnout.

Of course, at 372 pounds I wasn't able to do many of the activities to start but as I progressed and shed the pounds the variety of activities increased and kept me motivated. There are many physical activities to choose from:

- Walking, Jogging, Running and Hiking
- Biking/Cycling
- Lifting Weights & Using Weight Machines
- Exercise bands, exercise balls, medicine balls & kettlebells
- Cardio machines: Elliptical, Treadmill, Stair Climber, Stationary Bike, Rowing Machine
- Exercise Classes: Zumba, Dance, Spin, Step Aerobics, Yoga, Balance, Tai Chi
- Exercise DVD's
- Mini Trampoline
- Tennis, Pickleball, Volleyball, Racquetball
- Swimming, Water Aerobics, Water Zumba
- Ice Skating
- Skiing – Downhill & Cross-Country

- High Intensity Interval Training
- Circuit Workouts
- Boot Camp
- Pilates
- Climbing stairs, rocks or mountains
- Dancing, Line Dancing, Latin Dancing, Jazz
- Kickboxing
- Canoeing, Rowing, Kayaking
- Golf (walking – no golf cart)
- Jumping Rope
- Gardening/Yard Work
- Housework
- Washing the Car
- Add your favorites to my list

As I did with the diet side of the weight loss equation, I wanted to take bold steps with my exercise routine to ensure success. I put together a list of exercise tips that I followed and added to in route to my goal:

Exercise Tips:

#1 Hydrate with water frequently

#2 Do both cardio and strength training

#3 Start slow, 3-4 times a week for a month to ease into a routine and lessen the likelihood of injury or burnout. Then increase to 5-7 days a week taking no more than one day off at a time.

#4 Do a variety of exercises to help stay on track

#5 Choose types of exercises that I will stay with long-term

#6 Be sure to include stretching every day after exercise

#7   Do core & full body exercises to burn more calories (yes, that means squats and lunges, yippee!)

#8   Switch-up intensity level throughout cardio routine to increase the calorie burn

#9   Remember to breathe

#10 Exercise first thing in the morning – to keep from cancelling as the day's schedule changes. Early morning exercise will also boost metabolism all day.

#11 Lay out exercise clothes the night before so I see them first thing in the morning

#12 Challenge myself. Improvement is critical and motivational. Work for my personal best.

#13 Move to music – create playlists of upbeat music to keep a brisk pace while walking, jogging, stairclimbing, etc.

#14 Tunes not talk – music keeps the beat going whereas talking can slow me down

#15 Focus on my workouts. DO NOT look at emails, text messages or social media. DO NOT read books and magazines or watch T.V. while exercising. These distractions will slow me down, potentially cause injury and ultimately decrease my positive results.

#16 Wear good sneakers, alternate with pairs each day and replace every 6-9 months – or sooner if warranted

#17 Get fun, bright exercise clothes – look good, feel good!

#18 SMILE – often!

#19 Do a minimum of 45 minutes of cardio exercise 5+ days a week and do weight training 2-3 days a week. Use this format as my consistent plan so when deviation occurs I can easily get back on track. By being consistent I am building my new normal.

#20 When lifting weights – shorten rest time between sets

(15-30 seconds). As I progress, increase the number of reps & sets and increase the weights.

#21 Don't lift more weight than I can handle - must maintain good technique to reduce risk of injury and to get the positive results I am after

#22 Lift weights to full extension and return slowly to starting position, increasing muscle strength

#23 Don't lift weights 2 days in a row – muscles need time to repair

#24 On weight-lifting days do cardio exercise after my weight workout for greater fat burn

#25 Have FUN!

#26 Track activity – use an online tool/app or create a tracking chart (see example that follows *Tips*). My workout log shows how far I've come and continues to motivate me keeping the focus on what I am doing and can do.

#27 Don't compare my workout to others. Focus on growing my own confidence. If I am comparing my ability to others it could have a negative effect. A bit of competition is motivational – but beware of a defeatist attitude.

#28 Don't copy what others are doing in the gym unless I am sure they are doing the exercise correctly

#29 Alternate intense workouts with lighter workouts – change-up frequency, time and intensity – keep my body from getting used to the exact same activity which could slow down or stagnate the result/benefit

#30 Be flexible with workouts – a short workout in a busy schedule is better than skipping a workout day. Or fit two mini workouts into a busy schedule.

#31 If in pain – stop that specific exercise for a few days to a week. Use ice packs, take ibuprofen if needed, and do stretching exercises. I learned that if I didn't follow this regimen both the pain and down time would last much longer, causing anxiety about the potential delay in losing pounds. Continue to do cardio and weight training that doesn't affect the problem area.

#32 I am in the gym to workout not socialize. It is okay to let people know this when they are interrupting my routine, I am not being rude.

#33 Warm-up before cardio or weight-lifting

#34 Maintain good posture with all exercise

#35 Dance! It improves balance, coordination, flexibility and it builds stamina. Plus – it is a lot of fun!

#36 Stand tall when walking (don't lean forward) – look at the horizon or approximately 20-30 feet in front of me, to prevent back pain and bad posture

#37 Asphalt is a better surface than concrete (sidewalks) for walking & jogging. Concrete is harder which makes it worse for my arthritic joints and my muscles. But be careful if walking on a road, stay off busy streets!

#38 Change-up my regular walking by: walking briskly, adding some jogging, varying intensity, walking up and down hills, moving/swinging my arms, practice deep breathing, etc.

#39 Use a pedometer to track total steps per day – minimum of 10k steps

#40 Get in the car and drive various routes, loops and neighborhoods to map-out and measure distances that I can walk starting and ending at my door. Starting from home eliminates excuses. Changing up the "view" and the distance will keep me interested and motivated.

#41 Count down rather than up (3-2-1 instead of 1-2-3) with weights and exercises; on cardio machines change settings to elapsed time. Activities will seem to go by faster this way... it works!

#42 Work on balance to strengthen core

#43 Don't work out on an empty stomach; if hungry during a walk or workout eat some natural almonds, walnuts or pumpkin seeds

#44 Focus on the benefits of doing the exercise

#45 Use self-talk to motivate – "I can do this", "I am strong", "Way to go, Sheila!"

#46 Increase exercise effort as I get used to current length of time, distance, speed, steps, weights, reps, etc.

#47 When exercising – give it my all from start to finish

#48 At the end of each workout – ask: "Did I give 100%?"

#49 When finished with my workout praise my efforts and progress

Additional tips to support physical activity:

#50 Take the long way from point A to point B for added calorie burn; park further from destination

#51 Whenever possible – take the stairs

#52 At the office – set an alarm every 30-45 minutes to get up out of my chair and walk around

#53 At lunch time, when possible go for a 30 minute walk

#54 Pack gym shoes and exercise clothes for business trips and vacations

#55 Take an "Active" vacation (Country Walkers, Backroads, VBT, G Adventures, The Wayfarers.)

#56 Take a Spa vacation (Canyon Ranch Spa, Lake Austin Spa, Red Mountain Spa)

#57 Add outdoor fun physical activities as an alternative to the exercise routine

#58 Massage muscles

#59 Pamper my feet: foot soak, foot rub, pedicure

#60 Squeeze a stress ball

#61 KEEP MOVING! Burn more calories per day than I consume.

#62 Be patient, change takes time. Don't give up!

I created these lists with many exercise options and tips, and I used a variety of them, but the number one form of exercise I did consistently was (and still is) walking outdoors. Yes, walking does work. Walking is free and it can be done anywhere at any time.

You can lose weight by walking and eating a healthy diet. I am proof. I lost my first 50 pounds by walking and eating healthy before adding any other exercise activities. I feel great after walking (that happy feeling from endorphins) and I am pleased with accomplishing every step I take toward reaching my health fitness goal.

I used the exercise log (that follows) to track all of my fitness activities. While I didn't log my distance on the chart, I did measure my distance against time for most walking, jogging and cycling activities. Measuring distance to time was a good tool to show improvement. In the beginning it took me 25-26 minutes to walk a mile. Now depending on weather conditions and how far I am walking, I walk a mile in 15-17 minutes; slightly better than that if I add a bit of jogging. I'm no speedster but I get the job done.

EAT LESS + MOVE MORE = WEIGHT LOSS

Example of an Exercise Log

Daily Exercise Log   Month: <u>September</u>

Day of Month	# of Glasses of Water	Minutes of Stretching & Conditioning	Minutes of Weight Training	Minutes & Distance Walking & Jogging	Minutes on Treadmill, Mini Tramp or Elliptical	Minutes & Distance on Bike or Sta. Bike	Minutes of other Exercise (Zumba, Dance, Tennis, etc)	Total Minutes
1	9	10m	61m	42m	30m			143m
2	8			49m			50m	99m
3	7	10m	61m	41m	25m			137m
4	7			84m				84m
5	8	8m	54m			86m		148m
6	8	5m		117m				122m
7	8							
8	9	8m	66m	40m	36m			150m
9	10			99m				99m
10	8	5m	60m					65m
11	8			85m				85m
12	7		66m			63m		129m
13	8							
14	8			76m				76m
15	9		71m		20m			91m
16	10	5m		46m			50m	101m
17	10	10m	67m		30m			107m
18	8			53m				53m
19	8	7m	62m	49m				118m
20	7							
21	6			89m				89m
22	8	8m	63m		50m			121m
23	7					61m		61m
24	9	8m	67m	43m	25m			143m
25	10			42m				42m
26	8		71m		35m			106m
27	8	10m		91m				101m
28	7							
29	9	10m	62m	42m	30m			144m
30	9	7m		45m			50m	112m
31								

Days Exercised: 26   % Days in Month Exercised: 86.7   Avg Min per Day Exercised: 106.2m

Practice Positive Self-Talk

I am not perfect and that is okay. Yet, I have perfection within me, we all have perfection within us: from qualities and characteristics to skills, abilities, and intelligence. That is where I chose to focus.

Why are we so hard on ourselves? We waste too much energy on our less than perfect aspects. It's silly and serves no worthy purpose. Whereas, if I focus on my positive attributes I am much more likely to attract an optimistic and confident outcome, reaching my diet and fitness goals.

To improve my attitude I had my mantras in place to start each day, then with this step, I took building a positive attitude further. Positivity! I knew that when I am in a good mood I am energized and those good feelings and energy have a positive effect on my body and well-being. I wanted more of that.

I was open to achieving my objective when I pushed negative thoughts and words from my mind and let go of the "old stuff." By practicing positive self-talk I was giving me the energy and determination to succeed:

- When preparing a meal I praise my effort to fuel my mind and body with nutritious and beneficial food

- At the start of every workout I praise myself for making time to exercise and for understanding how important it is to take care of my health
- At the end of every workout I praise myself for working hard, for giving it my best, or for reaching a new target
- When I am weighing-in I praise my success; if there is a gain I remind myself of what I have accomplished and I provide encouragement for the week ahead
- I no longer look in the mirror and find fault. I look in the mirror and state, with a smile, "I like what I see!"
- I focus on positive reinforcements: "I can do this", "I am strong", "I am good", "I am worthy", "I am successful", "I am proud of myself", "I like who I am"

When we look at our own history, it is amazing how direct the correlation between our attitude and self-talk is, with the energy and fitness level of our mind and body.

We praise our family, friends, co-workers and even strangers. We show appreciation and gratitude to people in our lives and we feel awesome when we our given praise and shown appreciation by others (more on this in Chapter 9 *Gratitude.*) Surely we must have the capacity to cheer for ourselves, as well.

No sense in wasting another minute on self-negativity, give yourself a pat on the back, along with the praise you have earned! Be confident.

EAT LESS + MOVE MORE = WEIGHT LOSS

Educate & Equip

To aid my weight loss effort, to enhance my results and to build a healthy lifestyle long-term I continue to educate myself about:

- Improving fitness capability
- Enhancing flexibility, balance & posture
- Building endurance
- Building muscle strength
- Weight loss tips
- Solutions for sports injuries
- Researching best foods to boost metabolism and lower cholesterol
- Living a healthy life
- Low carb snacks
- Satisfying a sweet tooth in a healthy way
- Scrumptious healthy recipes
- Ways to burn more calories
- Finding healthy solutions to deal with stress
- Reducing the potential risk of diabetes, heart disease, cancer and other diseases
- Keeping my mind sharp and focused
- Improving my memory
- Living a positive life
- Learning a new sport/physical activity
- Etc.

There are many resources to use to gain this knowledge:

- Articles — Health, wellness, fitness and food articles in magazines, newspapers and online

- Books — Many book choices on health, diet and fitness to choose from. Check on Amazon.com or at your local book store.

- Magazines — Eating Well, Shape, Fitness, Health, Women's Fitness, Women's Health, Men's Fitness, Men's Health, Prevention, Self, Oxygen, Muscle & Fitness

- Websites, Apps & Blogs — Fitness.com, SparkPeople.com, Fitday.com, SnapFitness.com, ShapeFit.com, EatRight.com, BestFoodFacts.com, DailyBurn.com, Fooducate.com, Nutritioulicious.com, etc.

- Speakers — Health Clubs, Libraries, Church Groups, Local Hospitals, Associations, Media, etc.

- Trainers — Group and individual training is great for:
  - Learning how to use equipment
  - Learning correct techniques to avoid injuries
  - Explaining best practices for various exercises
  - Providing motivation and support
  - Giving feedback and praise

- Weight Loss Groups   Weight Watchers, SparksPeople.com, TOPS, WeightLossBuddy.com, PeerTrainer.com, Overeaters Anonymous, Jenny Craig, etc.

Take advantage of the many experts available through these resources. Put their expertise to practice daily; knowledge is golden.

To enhance my exercise capability and results I have used several of the following tools and equipment:

- Tools   pedometer, safety light, water bottle, bike helmet, fitness GPS, weight lifting gloves, knee & arm wraps, ice packs, callus removers & cushions, heating pad, stress ball, etc.

- Equipment   exercise band, jump rope, fitness ball, medicine ball, yoga mat, weights (dumbells), weight bench, kettlebell, mini trampoline, bike, cardio machines, step platform, workout bar, balance board, etc.

- DVD's   Walking fitness, Dance fitness, Zumba, Jazzercise, Yoga, Step Aerobics, Strength training/weights, (Denise Austin, Leslie Sansone, Tracy Anderson, Jilliam Michaels, Kathy Smith to name a few)

- Active Wear   gym shoes, tee shirts, exercise tops, exercise shorts, capris and pants, sports bras, bike shorts, hoodies, swim suits, socks, headbands, caps, outdoor gloves

- Other   scale, exercise charts, iPod/Shuffle or similar & playlists, etc.

EAT LESS + MOVE MORE = WEIGHT LOSS

Strategy · Step 6

Manage Social Events

Managing how I dealt with social activities and events was very important to achieving my weight loss goal short-term, and to living a healthy lifestyle, long-term.

So many activities and events include food and beverage:

- Holidays
- Birthdays
- Weddings
- Showers
- Graduations
- Anniversaries
- Retirement Parties
- BBQ's
- Pool Parties
- Picnics
- Happy Hour
- Game Night
- Club Meetings
- Conventions and trade shows
- Going out to Breakfast, Brunch, Lunch or Dinner
- Sporting events and tailgating
- Fairs and Festivals
- Going to the movies
- And more

While attending any one of these events it can be difficult to stay on track when:

- The food looks awesome
- The food smells incredible
- Attendees/Guests are praising how the food tastes
- I'm hungry and getting hungrier
- I don't want to insult the host/hostess
- My willpower is waning

I created a list of tips to help me through the food component of these events and still have fun:

Social Event Tips

#1 There are usually healthy food choices at most events – focus on those

#2 Eat something healthy at home before going out to curb my appetite

#3 Don't feel guilty saying no when offered unhealthy choices – I'm not offending anyone, I am being true to myself and my goal

#4 Drink plenty of water to feel full

#5 If consuming alcohol – stick with something lower in calories – and limit the number of drinks

#6 Fill-up on veggies and fruit – but skip the accompanying dips and sauces

#7 Choose lean protein – skip the sauces

#8 Resist temptation – don't graze at the buffet table

#9 Stay away from calorie laden appetizers

#10 Focus on the people not the food

#11 Participate in any activities to move focus away from

the food

#12 If invited to someone's home for a meal – offer to bring something. Make it a healthy option.

At Restaurants:

#13 Choose a restaurant with healthy cuisine or at least one that offers heathy food choices on their menu (check the restaurant website & their menu ahead of time)

#14 Don't go to buffet style restaurants

#15 Split a meal

#16 Once seated ask the server not to bring the bread basket or other included appetizer to the table

#17 Skip the appetizer if ordering a separate main course

#18 Order an appetizer or salad for my main course

#19 Order dressing on the side or no dressing if eating a salad

#20 Ask for grilled or steamed veggies with no butter or sauce

#21 Ask for a double order of veggies and eliminate the potatoes or rice

#22 Choose grilled fish, poultry or lean meats with no sauce

#23 Eliminate the bun or bread or at least the top half from burgers and sandwiches

#24 Ask the waiter/waitress to put half my entree in a doggie bag at the start of the meal

#25 Skip dessert or order fresh fruit

#26 Limit alcohol

EAT LESS + MOVE MORE = WEIGHT LOSS

Strategy · Step 7

Emotional Trigger Solutions

There will always be good days and days that fall short, the yin and yang effect. I needed a plan to help me through those days that fall short. I was an emotional eater and changing my behavioral responses to emotional and stressful situations had always been a difficult challenge. Old habits do die hard.

Paramount to my success was paying attention to the triggers and finding new ways to manage through them. This is where I have faltered and failed in past weight loss attempts and it's where I again faltered this time, which I detail in Chapter 10 *Conquering Setbacks*.

Stopping my automatic response to negative emotions and stress would take maximum concentration, effort and strength. I needed to live in the moment, mindful of what I was feeling and how I was going to respond to those feelings. This was my primary battle and it was crucial that I cure the emotional eating habit for good. It wouldn't be easy and would require repeated attempts. I simply needed to keep trying, again and again, until it became my new habit. I would not give-up. This would not defeat me.

I put together a trigger tip list I referred to when emotional or stressful pressures struck. It has helped on numerous occasions:

Trigger Tips:

#1   Be mindful – ask: "What am I feeling?"

#2   Concentrate on taking several deep breaths before reacting

#3   Slowdown and count to 10 (or 20, or 50...)

#4   Be mindful – ask: "How am I going to deal with these feelings?"

#5   Wait 15 minutes before responding to the feelings and urges to eat something unhealthy

#6   Smile – impact my mood immediately

#7   Go for a walk in nature

#8   State mantras and affirmations

#9   Do some cardio

#10 Go for a bike ride

#11 Lift weights

#12 Listen to or play music

#13 Sing – belt out a tune

#14 Dance – go wild

#15 Meditate

#16 Talk with a friend

#17 Call a family member

#18 Hug a friend or loved one

#19 Read a book

#20 Write

#21 Watch a movie

#22 Immerse myself in or take-up a new hobby

#23 Find a distraction: update social media, check emails, pay bills, etc.

#24 Take a bubble bath or soak in the spa/hot tub

#25 Watch a sitcom and laugh!

#26 Always have healthy snacks on hand – fruit, veggies,

nuts, yogurt – ready to grab when the overwhelming feelings attack

#27 Drink a cold glass of water

#28 Chew a piece of gum

#29 No sweets or chips in the house

#30 Brush my teeth & rinse with mouthwash, to keep from ruining fresh breath with food

#31 Repeat after me, "Don't sweat the small stuff"

#32 Be joyful

#33 Have faith... this, too, shall pass

#34 Be kind to myself

EAT LESS + MOVE MORE = WEIGHT LOSS

Strategy – Step 8

Support

While my weight and fitness goals are my responsibility, being able to discuss ideas, challenges, setbacks, and successes with family, friends, and others was an essential component. I was facing a big challenge and it was important to know I could count on others to encourage my efforts. I was very fortunate.

Their support helped in many ways:

- As a Cheerleader
- Sharing new weight loss ideas
- Providing weight lifting tips
- Camaraderie in exercise classes
- Empathy to the struggles and setbacks
- Providing a needed hug or kind word – encouragement
- Boosting my motivation
- Providing friendly competition
- Sharing healthy recipes
- Celebrating

I wasn't in this alone and that was immeasurable.

Appreciate and accept the kindness of others. Their support is an important component to achieving your goals.

EAT LESS + MOVE MORE = WEIGHT LOSS

Strategy – Step 9

Accountability

For me to attain this lofty weight loss goal would require drive, discipline, and grit. The best way for me to stay on track was accountability. I needed to be accountable to my goals, actions and results.

By measuring or tracking my activity I would be able to:

1. Chart my progress
2. Analyze my efforts
3. Determine diet and fitness changes I could make to improve results
4. Refer to my overall progress to spur me on when I hit a plateau
5. Cheer success on a regular basis
6. Reward achievement
7. Provide inspiration

I captured information at the start of this challenge that was valuable in aiding accountability and evaluation of my efforts. There were also a couple of things I wish I had captured at the start which would have provided additional ways to measure my success.

The Starting Point:

- Stats:
    o what I weighed

- o my body measurements – I wish I had taken my measurements at the start which would have provided additional encouragement as I progressed through the process
- Before photo – I should have taken a full-body photo when I got started, again for big impact. I didn't think of this until after losing over 100 pounds. As I hated to have my picture taken it was hard to find one at my heaviest weight, but not impossible.
- Keeping a pair of jeans in the largest size I wore to compare the size reduction. This had a very positive affect.

The basis of my accountability was monitoring progress:
- My starting weight – 372 pounds
  - I weighed once a week on the same day & time
  - I kept a chart of the results which provided on-going motivation
- Daily Food Consumption
  - I maintained a monthly chart/log (example page 47) that captured what I ate each day:
    - # of Calories
    - Fat grams
    - Protein grams
- Exercise Activity
  - I maintained a monthly chart/log (example page 56) that captured daily exercise activity:
    - Type of activity
    - Time
    - Distance (if appropriate)
  - In addition I monitored;
    - Steps taken

- Variations to cardio routines such as increasing speed and incline on the treadmill or increasing resistance and incline on the elliptical machine
- With strength training – I tracked and increased the number of pounds I lifted and the number of reps and sets I was doing

---

As stated in Step 5, *Educate and Equip* I chose to create my own charts for tracking, however, there are many good APPS and tracking gadgets to use:

- Fitbit
- Fitness Buddy
- My Fitness Pal
- Lose It
- Fitocracy
- Fooducate
- My Food Diary
- Calorie Counter PRO
- Jawbone
- Misfit
- Garmin (vivo-smart, vivo-fit, vivo-active)
- Cardio Buddy

I faithfully updated my food and exercise charts on a daily basis. The charts were a quick view of the current day against past days. *Was I on target? Did I need to make any changes?* The charts provided motivation, inspiration, and gratification, a winning combination.

I didn't use a trainer as I had a lot of exercise and weight-lifting experience. Although, being accountable to a trainer or to a workout friend would have been beneficial, too, as I would have been motivated to show-up and not let them down.

EAT LESS + MOVE MORE = WEIGHT LOSS

A year from now you will wish you had started today.

Karen Lamb

Chapter 6

Motivation

How would I motivate myself for the length of time it would take to lose 200 pounds? Just the thought of the immense task was overwhelming.

I would start with:
- **One day at a time**
- **One mile at a time**
- **One pound at a time**

It was day one and I was ready. (Refer to Chapters 2-5.) I went through the refrigerator and pantry and threw out the food I knew was unhealthy, removing temptation – a clean slate. I put together a list of the healthy foods I enjoyed, healthy foods to try and I planned a menu of meals for the first week. Then I went grocery shopping.

Week one was a success with the food/diet effort. I lost four pounds. But, it would take a balance of both diet and exercise to win the battle for good.

The diet side of the equation was a straightforward mental challenge. If I could overrule my emotional eating habits I was half way there. I knew what I needed to eat: 1,200-1,500 calories a day of lean protein, veggies, and fruits to start. I knew if I tracked my food consumption daily I could measure results and revise as needed to work toward the end goal.

With the exercise side of the equation it would be both a mental and physical challenge. It would take a week before I took my first steps. As heavy as I was, walking was the only exercise 1 could do to start.

I finally got myself out the door but I didn't go very far. At 372 pounds I wasn't ready to run a marathon... I couldn't even walk a full mile! As out of shape as I was I didn't let that deter me. Don't let it deter you either. Once you take the first step you will be encouraged to take the next one.

While I was on target with the diet part of the equation, for the first 6 weeks I did struggle with exercise, first walking just 0.5 a mile a day. I went out the door 4-5 days a week and put one foot in front of the other, slowly increasing my distance from 0.5 to 1.5 miles. I monitored distance against time for every walk striving to do a little more each day.

At 6 weeks I had lost 21 pounds and that was a big motivator to keep going but it was also a reminder that I still had a long way to go. While getting started was a huge challenge the bulk of the challenge lie ahead. To keep motivated, I created a list of reasons/reminders of why I wanted to lose the weight and I created a list of actions to take, that would help keep me on target:

My Reasons to Lose the Weight:

- Improve my health
- Improve my attitude
- Increase my energy
- Improve my fitness level

- Improve my appearance
- Participate in activities I used to enjoy
- Eliminate use of blood pressure meds
- Reduce diabetes risk
- Have more appealing clothing choices
- To feel good

My Motivation Actions:

#1   Stay positive – choose to be happy

#2   Boost my enthusiasm with mantras

#3   Review my attributes, capabilities and accomplishments

#4   Practice positive self-talk, daily

#5   Keep stress in-check

#6   Educate myself on diet and fitness suggestions, ideas and benefits

#7   Track and review progress on my charts – assess achievements

#8   Check (✓) the days I exercise on my kitchen wall calendar as a daily visual reminder and check the days I maintain my daily calorie intake (1200-1500 calories) with a different color marker

#9   Mark goals with rewards

#10   Deep breathing exercises to clear my mind

#11   Socialize with friends that have similar aspirations for their health and fitness – gain knowledge and inspiration

#12   Update music playlists – great tunes motivate me to move

#13   Add a new fun fitness activity. I bought a bike. I hadn't ridden a bike in 30 years. I would beg to differ with the phrase "it's as easy as riding a bike." Let me just say – buying a helmet was a good idea! It took a couple of weeks for the comfort level to kick-in and now I enjoy riding every week.

#14 Go dancing – let loose, have fun burning calories

#15 Check the scale and remember my starting weight

#16 Put on the fat jeans to see and feel the body changes

#17 Visualize my end result

#18 Go clothes shopping for something in my newest, smaller size

#19 Donate my fat clothes – incentive to stay on track

#20 Try a new healthy recipe

#21 Accept mistakes or set-backs and move forward

#22 Think good thoughts before going to sleep – waking up in a positive mood

Motivation would be a daily ritual, there would be days I jumped out of bed to get out the door and walk and there would be days I wanted to hide under the covers. Dealing with those low days head-on was crucial to my success. I kept pushing forward.

The motivation reminders, actions, and results would keep my momentum going for a long time.

We are made to persist...
That's how we find out who we are.

Tobias Wolff

Chapter 7

Fortitude

I was off to a good start, 6 weeks and 21 pounds gone! I
had dropped 10% of the weight but I still had 90% to go.
Early in this journey there were many days that I thought
about how much I still had to lose and questioned if I could
persevere. It would take mental and emotional strength,
endurance and resolve to achieve my goal. Fortitude.

Again, one day, one mile, one pound at a time.

- After 6 weeks of walking 0.5-1.5 miles 4-5 days a week I
  continued to increase my distance up to 2.5 miles.
- 2 months in and I was down a pant size. Yeah!
- Week 10 and I conquered the 3 mile neighborhood loop.
  Progress!

The Holidays

Not long after I began my weight loss plan the holiday
season arrived. The period included Thanksgiving, Holiday
parties, Cookie baking, Christmas, a Wedding, New Year's
and my Birthday. Oh no, that was a lot of pressure in a 7
week period. Would I maintain my diet and fitness
momentum?

The Holidays have always been emotionally stressful for
me, triggering old memories and unresolved issues, and I

would need focus and hard work to keep on track. Thanksgiving came first, I had promised myself that if I didn't eat dessert at all from day one of my journey until Thanksgiving I would treat myself to pumpkin pie. I kept that promise and enjoyed every delicious bite!

After one piece of pie would I be able to go right back to the plan, eliminating all sweets or would I be unable to adhere to my diet and fitness routine and end-up with the typical holiday weight gain? Fist bump! I chose to stay on plan. I worked diligently at it, and it proved successful. It was not an effortless task with all the temptations of the season but it was well worth the effort.

My *motivation reminders* were kept close at hand during this period.

Staying faithful to tracking both diet and exercise activity every day helped keep me motivated. For the rest of the holidays and through my birthday in January I was able to say no to all the sweets and fatty carbs. I also maintained my walking regimen throughout.

The praise and support I received from family and friends during the holidays also helped me stay on track. I lost 10 pounds during the 7-week period. I knew I still had a long way to go and I couldn't let up. I was getting results and staying the course was vital to achieving long term success.

I kept increasing my walking distance and speed and I continued to be vigilant on the diet side of the equation.

At this point you may be wondering when I was going to do more than walk for exercise. Walking was working, along with the diet, but I knew I would need to add other forms of exercise to reach my weight loss goal and achieve fitness success. Plateaus and dips in my effort would come, variety was needed.

When would I start the strength training (weight or resistance training)? You might understand my reluctance. A big part of my overall exercise routine and health improvement would include building muscle through weight lifting, eventually, but I was just too embarrassed to go to the gym at the start. The agreement I made with myself was that once I had lost 50 pounds I would start lifting weights.

Sixteen weeks into my diet and exercise commitment I went to the gym.

As I did with walking, I began slowly using both weight machines and free weights (dumbbells); starting with smaller weights and fewer repetitions and sets. It felt so good to add strength training to my routine. Of course, in hindsight, I wish I had done it from the beginning. Lifting weights builds more muscle and more muscle means burning more calories. An important component to the diet and fitness challenge as well as a key action to minimizing the effect of the aging process.

It isn't necessary to go to a gym to do strength training exercises. Using exercise bands, tubes, balls and dumbbells at home will provide beneficial results at little cost. You can also use your own body weight for resistance exercise such as push-ups, sit-ups, chin-ups, squats, lunges, step-ups. These exercises can be done anywhere at no cost and will achieve a positive outcome.

In addition to no-cost cardio exercise (walking, jogging, biking) some low cost cardio options include exercise and dance DVDs, a step platform, a mini-trampoline and Zumba or dance classes. Another no cost cardio option would be to borrow DVDs from the library (if available) or exchange them with friends.

Over time, along with my outdoor walking, I began to use the treadmill and elliptical machines at the gym for more cardio variety.

Having an alternative to walking outdoors (inclement weather) is very important to maintain momentum. In addition to using a treadmill or elliptical machine other options include mall walking, walking-exercise DVD's, stair-climber machines or simply climbing up and down stairs at home.

Walking was still my top choice for exercise. I went out the door between 5 and 5:30 am 4-5 days a week walking from 2.5 to 6 miles each morning. Eventually I enhanced the walking with short intervals of jogging. I went to the gym for strength training 2-3 days a week, and I used the treadmill or elliptical after lifting weights. A full schedule indeed but very manageable (usually 45-90 minutes per day) and it was working, remember I had 200 pounds to lose and needed a serious workout routine. I felt great!

I rarely let the weather affect my outdoor walking routine. I still felt vulnerable to the potential for falling off the wagon if I didn't stay on target with the exercise plan. I was working toward a new lifestyle one that included exercise 5-7 days a week for the rest of my life. The more I kept to that routine the easier it would be to get back to it should something occur that derailed me for 2-3 days (illness, injury, family emergency, business trip, vacation.)

I tracked my activity daily and once a week I weighed myself. At the end of each week I could see the improvement the diet and exercise was making which was a strong incentive to keep going. At the end of 12 months I had lost 124 pounds. Yeah, I was losing weight every week! That was an incredible incentive to keep going, but, there would be days of frustration ahead.

It hit me hard when after 54 straight weeks of ounces to pounds lost, I had the first week of no loss. When the 2nd and 3rd week of no losses happened I was worried that I would fall under the pressure. Panic.

I needed to keep my head on straight, to persist and stay positive. Thankfully I had several months of data to look at for inspiration. Keeping track of my daily activity and weekly results was invaluable and the praise I received from family, friends and neighbors kept me motivated. My food and exercise charts affirmed I was doing all the right things.

Experts tell us we will hit plateaus. It is what we do during those periods that make the difference between losing the battle and victory.

I didn't come this far to lose the challenge. I made small changes to my diet and exercise to shake things up. I expanded my list of proteins I was eating and increased my veggie choices.

For added cardio variety I bought a bike and I took Zumba (Gold) classes. Then I added some new strength training exercises, rotated the order I did the exercises and increased weights, number of sets and repetitions. I did this with several weight machines and free weight exercises. These changes would challenge my muscles and break the plateau.

For the next 10 months my journey continued as I dropped pound after pound, yet... that would change.

Celebrate any progress.
Don't wait to be perfect.

Ann McGee-Cooper

Chapter 8

Celebration

Celebrate and reward achievements.

Small achievements/goals should be celebrated along the way toward reaching the ultimate objective. Those smaller goals give us a chance to recognize where we are and how far we have come. They help energize and motivate us to continue to strive for success.

With such an overwhelming goal to attain it was important that I celebrate smaller achievements along the way to keep me headed in the right direction. Funny, who thinks a 50 pound weight loss is a **small** achievement? It is a very big deal and definitely deserves celebration!

I celebrated several achievements on my journey toward successfully accomplishing my goal:

- Losing 25 pounds, 50 pounds, 100 pounds, 150 pounds, 200 pounds
- My six month and one year achievements
- Going off blood pressure medicine
- First time I could walk 2.5 miles, 5 miles, 7.5 miles and 10 miles at one time
- First time I could ride my bike 10 miles, 15 miles and 20 miles at one time
- Dropping each pant size

I wouldn't let people take my picture during most of my "obese" years. I didn't want anyone to remember me that way.... I was too embarrassed and, yes, ashamed. Fortunately (can't believe I said that) my brother did take two pictures of me when I was at my heaviest weight. (Thank you, Scott!)

The photos are a reminder of how far I have come and give me a great reason to celebrate. As I made progress I could refer back to the photos, especially if I was at a plateau, and/or had taken steps backward. The comparison provided strong motivation to continue.

Keeping a pair of jeans at my largest size was a good idea. To visually compare the decrease in sizes was another reason to celebrate! Going from a women's plus size 28 to misses' size 10 and 12 is still hard to believe. I haven't been these sizes since my mid-twenties. I may or may not get to a size 8 and I am okay with that. I am healthy and strong. I like my curves and even at my age, I still feel a bit sexy!

Once I made the list of interim goals that I would celebrate it was time to get creative with a list of rewards. Celebration activities and rewards varied in size by target I had reached.

Rewards included:

- Manicure
- Pedicure
- Facial
- Massage
- Clothes shopping for a smaller size

- Buying a new exercise outfit
- Buying a new pair of gym shoes
- Buying a bicycle to add variety to my exercise routine
- Buying a new book – I love to read
- Buying new tunes – to add to my exercise playlist
- Going to a movie
- A Spa Day
- A hike through a state or national park
- Taking a Spa Vacation
- Taking an Active Vacation
- Celebrating with a great bottle of Wine or Champagne

Rewarding yourself for a job well done is a smart action to take. It provides an opportunity to reflect on the achievements reached and it inspires forward momentum toward your ultimate goal.

How will you celebrate your awesome achievements?

To speak gratitude is courteous and pleasant,
to enact gratitude is generous and noble,
but to live gratitude is to touch heaven.

Johannes A. Gaetner

Chapter 9

Gratitude

When I began this weight loss and fitness challenge I didn't tell anyone at first. If I were to fail why set myself up for more embarrassment? It soon became obvious that I was losing weight. The feedback I received was powerful and for that, I have many people to be thankful to and grateful for:

Family and Friends

As I stated at the beginning of this book the encouragement and praise I received from family and friends was significant and meaningful. On days when my objective seemed impossible and I thought I would never reach my goal I would get their positive feedback which gave me strength and momentum. Thank you!

Neighbors and Acquaintances

I was, without a doubt, living in the right community to execute my diet & fitness strategy and to meet my goals. During the past three years I have had dozens and dozens of neighbors at Westbrook Village, an active adult (40+) community, stop me while out walking to compliment and congratulate me on my weight loss. Neighbors stopped me in the gym while lifting weights and even at the local grocery store. It was awesome! I am grateful for their generosity and warm-heartedness. Thank you!

Kindness

Through my setbacks, family, friends and neighbors continued to cheer me on. They lifted my spirits at just the right time. No one commented on the temporary weight gain (detailed in Chapter 10 *Conquering Setbacks.*) When it became obvious I had regained weight they provided more positive encouragement and they reminded me of what I had and could achieve. I am so appreciative of their many kindnesses throughout my mission. Thank you!

Inspiration

To be told I have been inspirational to others has been incredibly rewarding. I have had friends and neighbors tell me they began their own diet and exercise program after seeing what I had accomplished. Thank you for sharing your stories... my best wishes for your success!

Positive Benefit

It only takes a moment to express gratitude but the positive benefit in doing so is enormous. Through my transition to a healthy lifestyle I have incorporated living with gratitude. The positive impact of living with and expressing gratitude every day has been lower stress levels, a greater calm and a heightened sense of well-being.

If you challenge yourself to work on a self-improvement goal, know that you can count on family, friends and others to support you and cheer you on. You don't have to go it alone. By expressing gratitude to them and yourself you will experience the positive benefits gratitude brings.

*Acknowledging a mistake just means that you
are wiser today than you were yesterday.*

Kelly Ann Rothaus

Chapter 10

Conquering Setbacks

Forgiveness is such an important topic it needs to be re-emphasized. Especially in light of my significant weight-loss setback.

I had reached my goal. I lost 201 pounds in 22 months. Hoorah! It was an awesome achievement and I was proud of myself. Just 21 pounds to lose to reach my ultimate goal (although I knew these pounds represented the excess skin that would be difficult to lose). I was so close. I might reach my ultimate goal in less than three years.

I was happy, excited, thrilled at what I had accomplished and I began celebrating. Big time! Just one day, I could afford it, right? Even if I gained a couple of pounds I would take it right off, no problem. But it didn't stop there.

At this same time I had decided to make a career change. I quit my job to pursue creating a small business and writing this book plus the accompanying journal. Over the next several months as I began this new challenge there was excitement and intensity but also anxiety, worry, stress, and major self-doubt which all fed into my old ways. I thought I had conquered the bad habits of emotional eating for good, after all I had survived a couple of high-stress periods during the 22 months of weight loss but nonetheless, I had plunged right back in.

Subconscious sabotage strikes, again. *If I regained weight then I couldn't publish this book or launch my business and therefore I wouldn't fail at the new challenge.* Crazy I know. Apparently I gave no credence to my major weight loss achievement and was back drowning in self-doubt.

Comforting stress and anxiety with unhealthy food was my nemesis; it had been my negative response behavior for many years. I slipped, well, actually I took a mammoth fall. In 8 months I had regained over 40 pounds. After all the hard work and dedication how could I have let this happen?

I failed the test.

Turning mistakes into lessons.

This was a big dose of reality. Making a major lifestyle change after decades of living with my emotional food addiction was not easy! Changing my old ways permanently while coping with life's stresses was going to take dedication every day for the rest of my life.

Bottom line question: "Do I want to feel good, have energy and be healthy or do I want that slice of carrot cake/bowl of ice cream/bag of chips?" I needed to get back to mindful eating and fast.

You would think there can't be a positive in this situation — but there was. I was still exercising regularly, both cardio and strength training, 4-5 days a week. Although I had stopped filling in my food count chart I was still filling in my exercise chart every day. Exercise was my saving grace otherwise I might not have been able to stop the hemorrhaging. However, it was clear that I couldn't burn enough of the excess binge calories to keep from gaining the weight. There weren't enough hours in the day.

Lesson learned... the hard way!

A powerful reminder.

Sustaining significant weight loss cannot be done without adhering to and maintaining a healthy diet, in addition to regular exercise.

I knew what I must do, it wasn't a crisis, yet. I had the plan in hand that had worked for 22 months. I needed to follow the steps and stay the course long term:

- First step: Forgive myself. I was changing years of embedded bad eating habits that had long been chained to my emotions. This was a challenge, a test, a setback. I knew when and why I had detoured. I would get back on track. While I did regain quite a bit of weight, I did not regain all I had lost. Far from it. This setback was manageable.

- Second step: Check my attitude and commitment. I had stopped taking the time to state my mantras. It was a priority for me to get back in the habit of saying them out loud every morning. I needed to reinforce my *Commitment Goal Statement* and review my motivation reminders. It was also vital that I squash the negative self-criticism that had crept back in and get back to positive dialogue.

- Third step: Remember what I have accomplished and how I did it:
    - Review my diet and exercise charts and give praise for what I had learned and achieved
    - Compare the scale today from when I began my weight loss journey
    - Try on the old pair of plus size jeans for inspiration

- Fourth step: Make peace with myself and mean it. **Food is not my comfort.** Refresh my emotional trigger solutions and keep the list close at hand.

- Fifth step: **GET ON WITH IT!** What's done is done. Don't dwell on it. Move forward in positive motion. *Try again.*

I did just that. I got back on track with healthy eating and I increased my exercise routine to 6-7 days per week. With forgiveness, a positive attitude and dedication to my mission, living a healthy lifestyle was becoming a reality.

If you, too, have hit a roadblock in route to reaching your goal, forgive yourself and... **try again.** Please don't give up. Believe in yourself and you will succeed!

My "aha" moment.

While out on an early morning walk, stating my positive affirmations, working on conquering my weight loss setback, I felt it, from my head to my toes. My true "aha" moment. It was all finally very clear and real. The struggles, the hard work, the emotional moments and writing this book had all helped me break through.

This is what I wanted. I was on the right path, my path. By listening to and feeling my mind and body in that moment I knew I would not go backward again. No more feeling tired, embarrassed or depressed because of my weight. No more.

From my internal core to my external being I knew that choosing to be healthy and physically fit was how I would live every day for the rest of my life. Hallelujah!

Passion and satisfaction go hand in hand.

Nicholas Sparks

Chapter 11

Healthy Lifestyle Achieved

After six months back on track, I did it - 200 pounds gone for good! I took bold steps forward and some missteps along the way but ultimately I succeeded. My diet and fitness goals have been achieved:

- I lost 200 pounds
- I am following a healthy diet
- I am consistently exercising 5-7 days a week
- I have a lot more energy
- I am off blood pressure medicine
- I have reduced my joint pain
- The threat of developing diabetes is gone
- I am living an active life
- I have found healthier solutions to dealing with stress
- I have reduced my self-doubt, eliminated the self-criticism and have more confidence
- My quality of life is vastly better
- Bonus - I feel great and I am happy!

Healthy lifestyle achieved. I am proud of myself.

The changes I have made to my attitude, my diet and fitness through continued attention and effort are now a way of life.

Attitude

Positivity. I like the word. It automatically makes me smile. I smile a lot more now. It's the first thing I do when I open my eyes in the morning. My mantras are still in view on the bathroom mirror, the refrigerator and on my office wallboard and I continue to state them daily.

Yes, there are stressful days and negative emotions do penetrate from time to time but my coping solutions have been permanently changed.

Diet

I work at being a mindful eater every day. I utilize my emotional trigger solutions so that I don't stuff my negative emotions with high calorie, unhealthy foods. Well, there is the occasional sweet, but no daily sweets and they aren't consumed to comfort stress, sadness or boredom.

Eating healthy foods has become habit. My key staples are lean proteins, veggies, fruits, nuts and whole grains (in moderation). I look forward to challenging myself creatively with great tasting healthy recipes.

I still maintain a food log to keep me on track and plan to do so indefinitely. I am not as strict on my daily calorie count but as an active female I do try to maintain 1,500-1,800 calories as my daily average with the occasional splurge.

I continue to work on those last 22 pounds but know it may take surgery to remove the excess skin. Those remaining pounds are motivation not to back track.

Fitness

I am happy to say that three years after starting my exercise plan it has become an essential part of my life. Understanding the importance of regular exercise as part of maintaining a healthy body and mind is a significant component of my well-being.

Exercise is a euphoric experience, a satisfying healthy addiction when practiced in balance. It is an automatic part of my early morning routine. I am dedicated to continuing a regular exercise schedule for life. I still track my exercise every day which motivates me and gives me satisfaction. It is an essential habit for me.

Old Habits - Gone

I will not go back to old habits! *(A new daily mantra!)* Although there will likely be bumps in the road and tests to pass I have the tools and proven success to maintain my new healthy lifestyle.

I will continue to use the essential elements that got me here:

Forgiveness
Attitude
Commitment
Strategy
Motivation
Fortitude
Celebration
Gratitude

Lifestyle Goal

As mentioned in Chapter 4 *Commitment*, I have created a
Lifestyle Goal Statement to help me maintain my vastly
improved diet and fitness lifestyle. The statement reminds
me of what I have learned and accomplished and it reminds
me of my healthy living transition.

My Lifestyle Goal Statement

*I am proud of my weight loss accomplishment. I will take
all that I have learned about maintaining a good diet,
adhering to daily exercise, and practicing positive self-talk,
and use those lessons to live the healthy lifestyle I deserve.*

I am now living my best life. You can, too!

Take a bold step with your own self-improvement challenge
and **try again**!

The greater the obstacle,
the more glory in overcoming it.

Moliere

Chapter 12

Cheers to Your Success!

I hope my story will inspire and motivate you to reach your goals.

Whether you have 25, 50 or 100+ pounds to lose or a different self-improvement goal to achieve you can do it! With these essential elements to guide you, you are starting out on the right path to success:

Forgiveness

It all starts with forgiveness. Take the emotional burden off your back and take your first step forward.

Attitude

Whether your goal is diet and fitness improvement or another challenge, get positive. With the right attitude you will achieve fantastic results.

Commitment

Defining your goal and making a commitment to that goal is your foundation and what you will measure your success against.

Strategy

With your goal set you are ready to determine the strategy that will work best for you. Educate yourself. Is your strategy balanced, is it achievable? Can you measure your efforts?

Motivation

Throughout your journey remind yourself of your objective and why you are pursuing it. Put together a list of motivation tips to help you stay the course.

Fortitude

Believe in yourself. You have the emotional strength, endurance and resolve to achieve your goal.

Celebration

Set incremental goals and celebrate those achievements with special rewards and recognition. The incremental successes will spur you on to reaching your ultimate goal.

Gratitude

Be grateful for:

- Forgiving yourself
- Challenging yourself
- Getting started
- Achieving your short-term and long-term goals

- Recognizing and appreciating what you have accomplished
- The support and love from your family and friends

Whether you use these essential elements or create your own diet challenge strategy, please consider that to make a permanent lifestyle change:

1. The underlying reason one overeats must be uncovered, owned and resolved
2. Quick fixes are usually temporary, it takes time, dedication and hard work to achieve lasting results
3. Simplicity: burn more calories than you consume
4. Be kind to yourself

Now it's time to get started. You are ready. You can do this!

Believe in yourself and **try again**.

Cheers to your success!

Sheila

When the world says "Give Up",
Hope whispers "Try it one more time".

Unknown

Dear Reader:

To help you in your quest to lose weight and get more physically fit I have put together a journal: ***BOLD STEPS – Diet & Fitness Commitment Journal***, which is a workbook to help guide you through the essential elements to reaching your weight loss objective.

Strengthen the commitment to your goal by putting your words in writing. Bring your strategy to life. Measure your results and honor your achievements.

These essential elements are also a good formula to help you achieve other self-improvement goals.

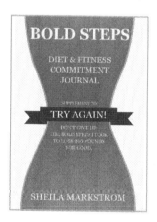

Your commitment journal is available on amazon.com or it can be ordered through your local bookstore.

Best wishes to you and your success!

Sheila

33206540R00068

Made in the USA
Middletown, DE
04 July 2016